"i can promi[se]
richey's interp[retation]
spirit ~ a [very]
thanksgiving d[ay]"

j. stone
www.jstonecards.com

❦

"Lisa is one of those rare, rare people who with a simple word, picture, quote, or thought touches deep into your soul, to that side that brings us from success into significance. She is a gifted guide on that journey."

Judy Girard
President, HGTV

❦

"It is an honor and joy to be a part of *Cheap Therapy*. There is an instant connection between the soul and the Truth! Thanks Lisa for spreading the word."

Fern
Fern's Garden
www.fernsgarden.com

❦

"I've enjoyed and been inspired by Lisa Richey's writings for years!"

Nancy Vince, President
Wholesalecrafts.com, Inc.
www.wholesalecrafts.com
www.acrelasvegas.com

༄༅

"Lisa Richey is the best combination of God centered spirituality, humor and gifted artist one can find in the modern world. Her "on-line" work and words on cheap therapy are the tip of the iceberg. Get the book and get the real thing.
The Rev. Margaret J. Neill, EdD
Priest in the Episcopal Diocese of East Carolina

༄༅

"Lisa is a breath of fresh air and a truly inspirational person to all who are lucky enough to know her. She has slain many dragons in her life and remains the most positive, optimistic role model anywhere in the world. Her grace allows people to embrace more of their whole self and her love of life is contagious. I pray Lisa writes her memoirs; I'm sure it would be a best seller! It should be titled 'How I embraced life in the face of obstacles, how MS gave new breath to me.' While MS can be a debilitating and devastating disease, Lisa has not allowed it to define her. Rather she has positively attacked MS with courage, an amazingly positive attitude, and a zest for life that is contagious."
Sue E. Thomas, President
Managing Asset Potential
www.MAPotential.com

Cheap Therapy
A Book of Healing Words

by Lisa B. Richey

Avar Press

ISBN: 978-0-9760660-1-9

Copyright © 2007 by Lisa B. Richey.

All rights reserved. No part of this text may be used or copied without written permission, other than brief quotes in the context of a review in whatever media, printed or electronic, or by whatever conveyance or storage device.

The photograph of Lisa B. Richey is used by permission of Tom Caperton.

Avar Press

Printed in the United States of America

10 9 8 7 6 5 4 3 2 1

This book is dedicated to Kendell L. Bearnes,

my dad.

1920-1983

Acknowledgements

Writing this message makes me MARVEL over how authors narrow their list of people to acknowledge. I don't want to omit anyone. So rather than have 42 pages listing the humans who've contributed to this book, I'll simply say –

If you've ever laughed with me; cried with me; told me your stories; listened to mine; sent me your poetry; shared beverages with me in my home; slept on my couch; bought Cheap Therapy; helped me believe when I couldn't; allowed me to believe for you when you couldn't; watched Life with me from a bench in silence; been kicked-out of any organizations or restaurants with me; diagnosed my body with M.S.; helped me slay dragons; helped me ride the dragons I couldn't slay; loved me; accepted my love; told me what I *oughta* do; given birth and strength to me *(and reminded me to wear my coat)*; been my BEST sister; or been the kind of unforgettable Life conspirator for whom there are no words – **I THANK YOU.**

Editor's Note

In *Cheap Therapy a Book of Healing Words*, Lisa Richey has penned a delightful set of inspirational thoughts. Numbering thirty-one, there is encouragement for each day of the month. Each is disarmingly simple, yet so basic for an enriched life. Curiously, all but a few are verbs, motivating the reader from her status quo. One exception is "normal," and Lisa clearly dispenses with the vagaries of *that* word. Another is "!WOW!" Well, that defines Lisa!

Her optimism, faith, and resilience will spur all of us to reexamine our lives and strive toward becoming better people. She will be remembered by children in the neighborhood, as is her current stated goal in her biographical information, but not for the reason she gave, in my opinion. Quite the contrary, she will be known then as she is now, as an indefatigable spirit who finds wonder in the simplest aspects of life and is grateful for the chance to give back to those less blessed than herself.

Contents

Author's Note i
Risk 1
Mend... 3
Learn.. 5
Ask 7
Forgive.. 9
Begin 11
Savor 13
Remember 15
Transform..17
Honor..19
Believe 21
Choose 23
Heal... 25
Flow 27
Declare... 29
Change..31
Listen 33
Treasure.. 35
Normal.. 37

Linger	39
Say	41
Ripple	43
!WOW!	45
Discern	47
Respect	49
Move	51
Drench	53
Be	55
Explore	57
Laugh	59
Balance	61
Cheap Therapy, the biz	63
About the Author	65

Author's Note

I've never believed the old adage that says "words can never hurt you." In my experience, words can hurt. They can also heal, encourage and inspire.

Words are powerful. That's why I do my best to choose them carefully. I don't always choose the best ones, but hey, I try.

Years ago I started making my own greeting cards because I couldn't find commercial cards that said what I wanted to say. That simple act ultimately prompted me to start a paper art business called Cheap Therapy. Cheap Therapy (the business) lead to this book.

Every month I send an e-newsletter to my customers, prospects, friends and family. As a part of those newsletters, I share a word that's meant a lot to me in the prior month, is guiding me as I step into the current month, or is just plain floating around in my brain. Hence, *Cheap Therapy: A Book of Healing Words*.

This book is a collection of 31 of my favorite words. We all know that many words have multiple meanings. I've explained how each of these words fits into my life and asked some questions about how they fit into yours.

There is no right or wrong way to read or use this book. Read it from cover-to-cover, all at once. Read a word a day, a week or a month. Start with page 1 or page 52 or page 36. Write notes or draw pictures in the margins (PLEASE)! This book belongs to you.

Here, let's make it official.

This book belongs to

_____

Thanks for buying *Cheap Therapy*. I hope you enjoy experimenting with it as much I enjoyed creating it for you.

Be well,

Lisa

Cheap Therapy
A Book of Healing Words

RISK

Risk giving up one thing for another that you value even more.

Take a financial **risk** on someone living a life you honor.

Take an emotional **risk** on something that reminds you to hope.

Take a spiritual **risk** on something that makes you say "!WOW!"

Assess **risk**s carefully and honestly. Then act accordingly.

Remember that you CAN have that one thing you want if you're willing to **risk** what you already have.

Risk your pride.

Risk your absolutes.

Risk your fears.

Risk being more even, more brilliant, more fulfilled than you ever dreamt possible.

Risk when you can't possibly resist **risk**ing. Remember that it's only when you can **risk** losing it all that you can **risk** HAVING it all… or at least having all that's worth **risk**ing.

༄

*For what are you willing to take your next **risk**?*

MEND

If you have things in your life that are torn, frayed or missing something—make the effort, **mend** them.

If *you're* feeling torn, frayed or like you're missing something—**mend** yourself.

Mend that part of you that allows too much of yourself to flow out—leaving nothing for yourself. **Mend** that stuck door on your heart and on your dreams.

Mending is about looking carefully and seeing the goodness within. It's about potential. **Mend**ing is about carefully placing together pieces that, at first glance, don't seem to match—but then—WOW!.

Mending involves not giving-up. It involves patience. **Mend**ing is not, however, about dwelling on something that's UN**mend**able. Let's face it, some things are beyond repair. So **mend**ing also involves discernment.

As you're **mend**ing remember that the only person you can **mend** is yourself. To others you make a**mend**s.

*What have you **mend**ed lately?*

*What do you need to **mend** next?*

What is stopping you?

LEARN

Pay attention to what you **learn** every day.

Make a list even.

Learn more today than you did yesterday.

Learn what you need to know. RE-**learn** what you didn't **learn** well enough the first time.

Learn what you want to know. REALLY **learn** what you didn't want to know. That way, maybe you won't forget.

Learn a language. Help others learn yours. **Learn** about trees, plants, birds, fish and flowers. **Learn** about music, movies, plays and (of course!) books!

Learn more about yourself by **learn**ing about others. **Learn** something new about that person who's left you breathless for years.

Learn even more about THAT PERSON whose very presence makes you cringe.

Once you **learn** something, teach it to someone else who wants to **learn** it, too.

And remember that as long as you live, you'll keep **learn**ing the very same lessons over and over and over until you've **learn**ed your REAL Lesson.

WHO KNEW?!

※

*What have you **learn**ed lately?*

*What do you **learn** over and over (and over and over...)?*

*How do you **learn** best?*

*What keeps you from **learn**ing?*

ASK

Ask for what you need.

Very few humans are mind-readers.

Fewer still are jerks who simply want to deny and hurt us.

So we must **ask** for what we need if we want any chance of receiving it.

Nothing ventured, nothing gained, aye?

Ask WHY?
Ask WHY NOT?
Ask HOW?
Ask HOW MAY I HELP YOU?
Ask WHY ME?
Ask WHY NOT ME?

*Why not **ask?***

*What do you need to **ask?***

FORGIVE

Experience the power of **forgive**ness.

Say *I **FORGIVE** you*, and
mean it.

Forgive everyone who ever wronged you, including yourself.

Forgive him for breaking your heart.
Forgive yourself for breaking his.

Forgive her for telling your deepest secret.

Forgive the people you love for not loving you back the way you want them to love you back.

Stop holding grudges and **forgive**.

Forgive yourself for being human, for not knowing all the answers all the time.

Once and for all, for the sake of your own sanity, **forgive.**

Ask for **forgive**ness. Accept **forgive**ness. Offer **forgive**ness.

For life, for love, for peace, forever, for them, for you **forgive.**

൚൨

*When were you last **forgiven**?*

*How did you accept **forgive**ness?*

*What will help you **forgive**?*

*Why not **forgive**?*

BEGIN

Start something.

Put one foot in front of the other and inch forward, even slightly.

Begin making progress instead of excuses.

Show up.

Say *Hello* and **begin** a conversation.

Say "*Says who?*" and **begin** a revolution.

Write one sentence and **begin** your novel.

Begin again. This time in a different key.

Begin putting yourself first. **Begin** enjoying it.

Begin an intentional community, if that's how you want to live.

Begin a reading group and focus on people who've made bold new **begin**nings.

Begin a new way of eating; a new way of moving; a new way of finding stillness and a new way of being at peace.

Begin as soon as you finish reading these words.

Begin at the **begin**ning and don't even think about where it will take you.

Now, **begin.**

༻❀༺

*What are you ready to **begin**?*

*What steps are you taking toward your **begin**ning?*

*What scares you most about **begin**ning?*

*What thrills you most about **begin**ning?*

SAVOR

SLOW DOWN and enjoy every taste, every smell, every smile, every experience.

Savor your life.

Savor your coffee (or tea) for at least forty-three minutes at least one morning each month.

Read that poem, letter, love note, card or e-mail you cherish word-by-word, letter-by-letter. Read it again even more slowly.

Give yourself thirty-six bites to finish your favorite chocolate bar.

Life isn't given to us to be gulped or gobbled. It's given to be tasted, lived moment by moment—in the moment.

Life is meant to be **savor**ed.

Savor your time with a child by giving one more twirl or story.

Savor yourself by taking two more moments of quiet.

Savor stories (especially when you've heard them before) along with the story teller.

Savor holy seasons.

Savor the people with whom you share those seasons. That perfect gift, table setting or party dress can all be returned. Humans can't.

You can't save a moment in time, but you can **savor** it.

༄༅

*When was the last time you noticed you were not **savor**ing?*

What did you do about it?

How will you prevent that from happening again?

REMEMBER

Remember who you are and from where you came.

Remember all the laughter and all the tears.

Remember the love and all the fears.

Remember how it felt the first time you kissed THAT someone full on the mouth. **Remember** the day you hoped would never end. **Remember** when it did.

Remember the first time you experienced something that left you feeling awe. **Remember** the last time that happened.

Remember where you were and what you were doing the first time you heard your all time favorite song.

Remember the first time you met your best friend.

Remember why she's still your best friend.

Remember the first time you met someone who helped you feel invincible. **Remember** the last time you helped someone else feel that same way.

Don't worry about not **remember**ing your complete schedule, grocery list or other people's e-mail addresses. We have calendars, to-do lists and address books for that stuff. **Remember** the important things instead.

Remember when someone you loved died and when someone you didn't even know died.

Remember when parts of you died—or when you put them so high on a shelf you couldn't reach them.

Remember your dreams. Now **remember** how to get them back.

༺༻

*Do you **Remember** when...?*

TRANSFORM

Realize that you change everything you touch. You are a **transform**er.

Transform yourself and notice how everyone around YOU is suddenly **transform**ed.

Transform your fear into faith, your confusion into clarity; and your judgment into love.

Transform your relationships with the people you love and the planet you love.

Transform your thoughts into action and your ideas into reality.

Transform that dark and dingy room into a light and airy space.

Transform that old, beaten-up trunk into something that holds magic.

Transform some leftover chicken and potatoes, half an onion and a few drops of olive oil into dinner for two.

Transform your used and worn out beliefs about your own limitations. Tune in to your powerful, one of a kind frequency and be the **transform**er you are.

ॐ

*What **transform**s you?*

*How were you last **transform**ed?*

*How did you last **transform**?*

*How will you continue to **transform**?*

HONOR

Honor yourself for the shiny and tarnished human you are. **Honor** other people's sparkles and stains, too.

Honor YOUR and other people's time. Invest and exchange both wisely.

Honor the people who tell stories; who remember the old ways; and who have time for the young.

Honor the people who fight for our country when war is called and the people who fight to stop war. **Honor** soldiers, sailors, airmen, protestors, leaders and their families.

Honor people who are riding the dragon of disease. **Honor** people who rode as long as they could.

Honor the people in your immediate world with your heart, laughter, tears, ears, hugs or a great cup of coffee and a pecan roll.

Honor the people who clean, repair, paint, govern, grow, preach, defend, protect, dig, hide and build.

Honor this earth and what or whomever you believe created it.

Honor who and what is in front of you as you want to be **honor**ed and accept their **honor** of you as it's offered.

❦

*What do you **honor**?*

How do you show it?

*What **honor**s you?*

*When did you last feel **honor**ed?*

BELIEVE

Believe in something bigger than yourself.

Believe in something, anything that will lend you hope, courage, and strength when your reserves are depleted.

Believe in fairy tales—remembering that *happy endings* is a relative term.

Believe what others tell you—when it rings true in your gut.

Believe what your gut tells you.

Believe in yourself.

Believe you are infinitely powerful, brilliant, beautiful and capable of changing the world.

Believe you me!

CHOOSE

Every moment of every day, **choose**.

Choose to fear less and love more. **Choose** to shout less and listen more. **Choose** to eat less and taste more. **Choose** to regret less and hope more. **Choose** to do less and be more.

Choose to live every day of your life.

Choose to respond with what you really think and how you really feel rather than how you think someone else thinks you SHOULD respond.

Choose the water over the soda.

Choose the lemon juice and olive oil instead of the blue cheese dressing *(at least once in a while)*.

Choose the walk around the block instead of the ride to the mall.

Choose simplicity over extravagance.

Choose conversation over television or I-pods.

Choose forgiveness—especially with yourself.

Choose to look at each other a few moments longer without filling the space with unnecessary words.

Choose to laugh out loud at least once a day.

Choose to make your own mistakes and **choose** to dive into their lessons.

Choose to accept other people's choices as their own.

Choose to make your own choices in your own time and **choose** to stick with them.

How

Will

You

Choose??

HEAL

Human, **heal** thyself!!

Once and for all, take off the band-aids of your emotional scars, psychic wounds, physical diseases and set about **heal**ing them.

Remember that you're not alone in your brokenness. We're ALL cracked in some way!

It's up to us to **heal** by talking, painting, creating, cooking, listening, dancing, singing, writing, reading, hiking or canoeing.

If it feels **heal**thy it probably IS **heal**ing.

Heal in solitude, in a group, in a doctor's office, in a circle, in a church, in an ashram, in a clinic, in a monastery, on the beach, by a lake or in the mountains.

Just let the **heal**ing begin.

Heal with the help of others you trust. **Heal** in 12-steps, or 367 steps or 1,200 steps. Just take the first step.

It's never too early nor too late to let the **heal**ing begin.

Heal with meds, herbs, energy, touch, exercise, yoga, tea, coffee, doctors, counselors, shamans, meditation or prayer.

Remember that **heal**ing arrives in countless and often surprising time frames, disguises and vehicles. Like most wonderful things in Life ~ **heal**ing often sneaks up on us.

Heal others by **heal**ing yourself. **Heal** your community by healing yourself. **Heal** the planet by **heal**ing yourself.

Heal!

ക

*From what are you going to **heal** yourself?*

FLOW

Go with the **flow.**

Why even try managing and planning your way through life? Amid the time clocks, deadlines, cell phones and beepers, life really can be a great ride. Why not enjoy it?

There is no need to fight the current. Remember that CURRENT = The PRESENT. Why fight that? It is what it is.

I'm not suggesting you allow yourself to become anyone's doormat. Just be open to the unplanned. Hey, you might as well because, well, you know what happens to many plans.

Sometimes, we just have to go with the **flow** and trust that something or someone wiser than us will handle the details.

Yep, go with the **flow.**

*How do you try to manage or plan the **flow**?*

*Has the **flow** ever been *better* than YOUR plans?*

*Why not try going with the **flow**?*

DECLARE

Declare your freedom.

Declare yourself in balance with others—no better and no worse; no wiser and no less wise.

Declare your support for other humans, for animals, for the Earth and for ones too often forgotten *(including yourself)*.

Declare your equality and independence.

Declare your wisdom and willingness to learn.

Declare your strengths and weaknesses.

Declare your attractiveness and quirkiness.

Declare your faiths and fears.

Declare your dreams and goals.

Declare your past and future as you're living your present.

Declare your love and limits.

Declare all of who you are.

And when you notice others **declar**ing who they are, say out loud (preferably with a slightly sassy twang and sizable sassy smile, as we do here in the South),

"Well, I **declare!**"

ೋೋ

*What did you last **declare**?*

*What **declar**ations have you heard lately that impacted your life?*

*What do you need to **declare** next?*

CHANGE

Be the **change** you keep hoping to see.

Be the **change** you keep waiting for others to be.

Change what needs **chang**ing**.**

Change what you can **change.**

If there are things that need **changing** and you can't **change** them—**change** your attitude.

Change your volume without **chang**ing your voice.

Change your vision, but not your values.

Change your vistas, but not the vitality of who you are.

*When making waves isn't enough . . .
make **change**.*

LISTEN

Listen loudly.

Be quiet and see how much there is to hear.

What are people saying and NOT saying? **Listen** to them.

If you're having trouble **listen**ing TO things—**listen** FOR them.

Don't just be an active **listen**er. Be a PRO-active **listen**er.

Listen to the last notes of every song. **Listen** to a sunrise. **Listen** to the sounds outside your home very late at night.

Listen to your gut. It really DOES make noises and they are wise noises. **Listen** to and for them. **Listen** for and to your God (whatever you call her).

Hear the dawn, the water, the crickets, the thunder, the soap bubbles and the encouraging voices.

Don't **listen** to the negative voices. They are not meant for You.

Listen to your body.

Listen with your body—your heart, head, eyes and even your ears, if necessary.

And always, *ALWAYS* **listen** to small print and what is between the lines.

༄༅

*On a scale of 1-10 (10 being best) how good are you at **listen**ing?*

How good do you WANT to be?

How will you get there?

When will you start?

TREASURE

Recognize what's important to you and **treasure** it. Whether it's a time of day, a certain place or person, a cup of coffee, or a favorite meal; if you **treasure** it —**TREASURE** IT.

Turn **treasure** into a verb rather than a noun. Make it something you DO—not something you hoard.

The next time you see something (or someone) you **treasure**—notice it carefully; as if THIS was the first time you'd ever seen it. Examine it closely as the priceless creation it is. Be in awe of what you **treasure**.

Say *(out loud)* "I **TREASURE** YOU."

Treasure the people with whom you can laugh, cry, learn and teach.

Treasure every moment, knowing it can never be replicated.

Treasure every lesson—*especially* the ones you didn't want to learn.

Treasure pixie sticks and lavender. **Treasure** how the birds and squirrels share the seed outside your window. **Treasure** music and books. When you really **treasure** something—share it with someone you **treasure.**

Treasure the sunshine and rain—the heat and the cold.

The next time you start to wish for something different, **treasure** that you can feel what's happening right now.

Take nothing for granted. **Treasure** everything that helps you find your way.

୨୦୧

*Make a list of all that you **treasure**.*

If your list is shorter than you'd like -

GO

ON

A

TREASURE HUNT.

NORMAL

Normal is just a setting on the dryer.

In most of the real world **normal** doesn't exist. So be something that does. Just don't be **normal**!

Be yourself.

Be brave.
Be afraid.
Be loud.
Be quiet.
Be coy.
Be bold.
Be blonde.
Be brunette.
Be red.
Be gray.
Be purple, even.
Just don't be **normal**!

Normal isn't TRUE.

Normal just isn't what it's cut out to be.

Start something new and healthy. Stop something old and unhealthy. Forget seeking **normal**cy.

Why wish for **normal** times? Have you ever really had any? When you're hoping for **normal**, you're missing what IS. And what IS—is always what's most important.

Be exactly who, what, when, where, why and how you are. And the next time you find yourself longing for **normal**—go look at your dryer.

∞

*Why is **normal** so important to you?*

*When did you last feel good about being **normal**?*

*How has NOT being **normal** helped you?*

*How will you celebrate NOT being **normal**?*

LINGER

SLOW DOWN.

Yes, time is limited.

There's so much that absolutely, positively MUST happen. AND every single moment we're alive is irreplaceable.

Honor each one by **linger**ing with it.

Sip the last drops of your tea instead of gulping them. Finish your conversation before running to the next item on your calendar. **Linger** at watching the person singing in the car next to you at the stoplight, the young man clearing the restaurant table next to you, the child practicing for the pageant. **Linger** with the memory of That Kiss.

If you're at a party, **linger** there, rather than anticipating the NEXT ONE. You never know, you might find something (or someONE) you want to **LINGER** with.

Look at the sky a bit longer before you get into your car. Pick a leaf of rosemary or lavender and before continuing on, rub it between your fingers and **linger** over how beautiful it smells. It doesn't matter how long it will take for you to get TO your vacation spot if you're not living until then.

Linger as you listen *(especially when you've heard the story many times before)*. **Linger** over coffee. **Linger** at the grocery store. **Linger** over dinner. **Linger** in bed. **Linger** as you create. **Linger** in the shower. **Linger** as you walk the dog.

And of course, **linger** longer with those you love.

అఎ

With what/whom will you now linger longer?

SAY

Say what you mean.

Say "*Thank you"* (for all kinds of things).

Say "THIS it what's important to me and this is what I'm doing about it."

Say "*I love you."* **Say** "*I love you, too"* or **say** "*I can't say that.".*

Say "*I'm sorry."* **Say** "*I'm sorry, too"* and **say** "*I forgive you.".*

Say "*I miss you."* **Say** "*It's good to know you've missed me."*

Say "*I need your help."* **Say** "*I can't help you this time."* Or say (if you MEAN it) "I would be happy to help you."

Say "*You hurt me."* **Say** "*I'm sorry I've hurt you."*

Say "*You're looking great.* **Say** "*I'm glad I look great to you.".*

Say "*Hello*" and then smile all the way up through your eyes.

Don't be afraid to **say** it before others do.

Say what you **say** through three filters:

Is it honest?

Is it necessary?

Is it loving?

Yep, **say** what you mean to **say** and then Trust.

⁓∾⁓

*How easy is it for you to **say** what's important to you?*

*How was it for you the last time you did **say** what you needed to **say**?*

*How will you do a better job of **say**ing what you need to **say**?*

RIPPLE

When was the last time you stopped to watch how far a **ripple** travels across water?

When was the last time you *started* the **ripple**?

Sometimes it's necessary to make waves. Often, a **ripple** will work. Unlike waves, ripples have great endurance rather than brute force. They also carry rather than crush.

Ripples whisper Transformation—rhythmic and encouraging.

Cause a **ripple**. Be a **ripple**. Notice **ripples**. Be carried by **ripples**. SAY **"ripple"** five times real fast. It's a GREAT word!

Think about someone you know who's started a **ripple** that's changed your life for the better. Now contact that person and thank him! Remember that no change in the world happens without a catalyst—without one small **ripple**. Rather than wait for someone else to make the change you want (*or even worse complain about it*) DO SOMETHING to make the difference you want. You'll be amazed how far your **ripple**s will travel.

Let's all be **ripple-**rousers**!**

*What was the last **ripple** that changed your life?*

*What was the last **ripple** you started?*

What will be the next one?

How will you let 'er ripppppppp?

!WOW!

If you haven't had a **!WOW!** moment lately, I hope you'll look for one today.

It's amazing how many of them are out there, if only you'll pay attention. Did you see that sunrise this morning? **!WOW!** If you're not a morning person, how about that sunset? **!WOW!** See? It's that easy.

Just look around you—children, pets, flowers, birds, strangers, people we've loved for years *and thought they could never **!WOW!** us again*, rainbows, answered prayers, even prayers that weren't answered the way you hoped… you name it. **!WOW!** moments abound. Claim them!

As I type this message, I'm watching a squirrel leap from a chair into the seed holder I have hanging from one corner of my home. He made it! **!WOW!**

One of the best things about **!WOW**! moments is sharing them.

I've always heard that a smile is meant to be shared. I think the same goes for **!WOW!** moments.

Commit to finding at least one each day and then tell someone about it.

You never know, you might become someone else's **!WOW!**

Let's all become **!WOW!**-mongers.

༄

What last helped you say !WOW!?

When did you last help someone else say !WOW!?

How do you go about finding !WOW! moments?

How do you encourage others to spot !WOW!s?

DISCERN

Make your own choices.

Discern with whom you want to spend time, in which relationships you want to invest and respond accordingly.

Hopefully there will be some time for YOU in your response.

Neither time nor energy is infinite. If you feel you've given away too much of either, remember who really holds the purse strings. Spend wisely.

Discern deliberately.

Take a moment. Take three. Heck, take TEN.

You **discern.**

What does your gut tell you?

What does your heart tell you?

What does your *inner ear* tell you?

What does your brain tell you?

Trust your ability to **discern** what's right for you and what isn't.

If the answer isn't
clearly YES!...
it's probably No.

ುಲ

*When did you last **discern**?*

*How do you **discern**?*

How do you know when you KNOW?

What gets in your way?

What now?

RESPECT

Respect is not a right. It's a privilege that's earned.

Earn the **respect** of yourself and others by living your own true life.

Extend your **respect** to others who are living theirs.

Respect the experience of others without negating your own.

Respect the awesome power of this Earth and all that is good—remembering that you are part of it.

Respect your body.

Respect others who respect theirs.

Remember that **respect**ing one thing or person does not require negating anything or anyone else.

Respect begets **respect.**

*What do you **respect**?*

MOVE

Move anything in your life that's rusty, stiff or stuck and get into motion.

Take a walk.

Take a hike.

Take a step away from stagnating jobs, relationships and life patterns.

Move into the life you are meant to be living.

Move closer to people who meet you with honesty and who help feed your wildest dreams.

Move away from everybody else.

Remember that you don't have to **move** mountains. Shifting a single pebble can work wonders.

Just **move.**

Make your **move** **any **move**** NOW.

If you wait until you have more money, time, security, patience, grace... more anything... you'll never **move** anywhere at all.

THIS is your time to **MOVE**.

※

*When was the last time you made an important **move**?*

How did that work out for you?

How did you know it was TIME?

How will you know the next time?

DRENCH

Drench with things that nourish.

Drench your cereal with more fresh fruit and less refined sugar.

Drench your garden with water and food.

Then **drench** your home with flowers, veggies and herbs.

Drench your imagination with books.

Drench your fear with faith.

Drench your wars with peace.

Drench your schedule with space.

Drench your presents with Presence.

Drench your day with laughter.

Drench your friendships with hearing.

Drench the children in your life with reminders that they matter to you.

Drench yourself the next time it's raining outside.

Drench the people you love with who you are.

Remember that **drench**ing is different from dipping in that it requires hope and confidence.

Be hopeful!

Be confident!

Be a dynamic **drench**er!

༄༅

*When was the last time you allowed yourself to be completely **drench**ed*

by a steady rain?

*If it's been more than ten years—**drench** yourself very, very SOON.*

BE

Be who you are.

Forget about trying to **be** anyone or anything you're not. That's a waste of precious time and energy.

If you're not sure who you are. Start **be**coming yourself.

It's great.
YOU'RE great!

Be where you are.

Stop imagining where you will (or think you NEED to) **be** in five minutes, five days or five years.

There is no time like the present.

Be there.

Be more and do less.

Be brave when you can.

Be true when you speak.

Belong when you want.

Beware when you react.

Behave when you must.

Begin **be**ing.

                        ﻖ୬

*What keeps you from **be**ing yourself?*

*What helps you **be** yourself?*

*When was the last time you caught yourself **be**ing someone else?*

How will you keep that from happening again?

EXPLORE

Be an **explore**r.

Don't just sight see—**explore**.

Get out of the car. Get out into the places you visit. Touch the trees. Taste the food. Hear how those birds sing. Hear the stories those people tell. See how that river flows. And dare I say it? Smell those roses.

When looking for someplace, something or someone—**explore** the less than obvious. **Explore** the obvious, too. How often is it that what we're looking for is right in front of us?

While you're **explor**ing, look in the mirror. Really look at that face. If you don't recognize who's looking back at you, get to know her or him again—maybe for the first time. **Explore** yourself.

Explore. And be sure to be ready. So when the time is right, you can shout "EUREKA! I found it!"

*When was the last time you went **explor**ing?*

When will be the next?

LAUGH

Laugh out loud every day.

Laugh at yourself as often as possible.

Laugh with others. Help others **laugh**.

Laugh 'til tears run down your cheeks.

Laugh 'til your stomach aches.

Laugh 'til your face hurts.

Laugh 'til you lose your breath.

If you can't remember the last time you **laugh**ed like this, LOOK for reasons to **laugh**.

Watch (and listen) to kids and animals.

Read a book or listen to music that lightens your load.

Look in the mirror and make funny faces.

Blow bubbles.

Lay on the floor with a group of friends. Put your heads on each other's stomachs and play the "Ha-Ha" game (remember THAT one)?!

Find someone who loves to **laugh** and follow their lead.

Remember that **laugh**ter really IS the best medicine.

So heal yourself.
Laugh.

༄

Find something to help you
laugh *out loud*
TODAY!

BALANCE

Life is all about **balance.**

Balance your work time with your play time.

Balance your social butterfly time with some quiet and solitude.

Balance your time with your kids with time with the person who's raising them with you. And hey, vice versa on all of these.

If you've been giving too much, let people know you're ready to receive.

Balance. If you always call them, let them know you'd love to hear from them.

If they always connect with you first, make a point to extend your hand first next time. Don't keep score. Seek b**alance.**

If you've been going at breakneck speed, slow down before an accident or your body does it for you. **Balance.**

If you've been sitting in front of a screen (ANY screen) too long, get up from your chair or couch and dance, walk, swim or just stretch. **Balance** your body.

When you feel you've been **balanc**ing too much for too long, put some things down. Please, do that carefully though. You don't want to lose your b**alance.**

ೞಲ

*What's out-of-**balance** in your life?*

*How are you going to regain and maintain your **balance**?*

CHEAP THERAPY, the biz.

Now that you've read *Cheap Therapy*, the book, you may be interested in knowing more about **Cheap Therapy, the biz.** It began in 2000, not long after I'd stepped out of a long banking career, due to the adventures of multiple sclerosis. I wanted to create something to donate to places I'd previously supported financially. To my surprise, people began contacting me to buy my stuff. That's when I realized this new adventure of mine needed a name.

I'll never forget sitting at the kitchen table of a dear pal (thanks Jackie Mc!), when she, one of her daughters (yay Sarah), and I realized that creating paper art would probably save me thousands of dollars in conventional therapy. SOOOOOO, **Cheap Therapy...** paper art that celebrates life, was born.

Cheap Therapy now creates for more than 800 art galleries, book stores and gift shops across the US. To date there are 11 part-time Cheap Therapists. That includes me, since I can only work at this adventure 10-12 hours a week. We create handmade paper, greeting cards, magnets, bookmarks, posters, journals and other handmade books in my home studio.

I work very hard at maintaining balance in my life and business. My intention for *Cheap Therapy*, Inc is to celebrate life. No one involved with Cheap Therapy is getting rich from it (financially, at least). The business pays for itself and at least 90% of our profit goes to various charities including Habitat for Humanity, the American Red Cross (disaster relief fund), the National Multiple Sclerosis Society, the Cheap Therapy Pay it Forward Grant, the Brownies and the National Honor Society. I was kicked out of these last two, so they hold a special place in my heart. If you'd like to know even more about Cheap Therapy—paper art that celebrates life, I hope you'll visit my website: www.cheaptherapy.net.

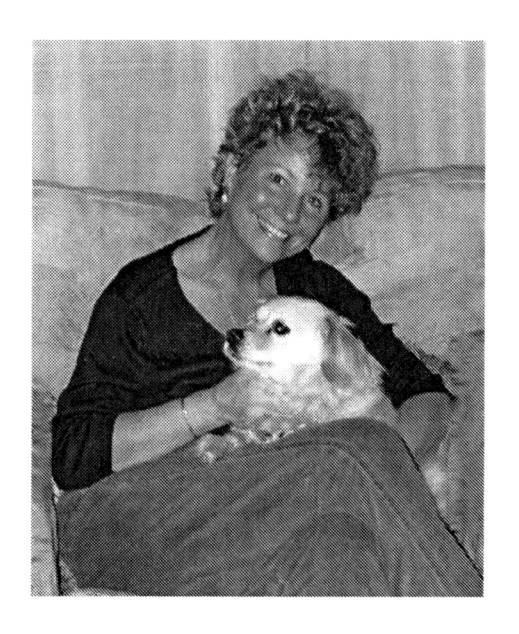

Lisa Richey is a North Carolina native. She grew-up in Havelock; had her first car wreck in Atlantic Beach; learned how to pick blue crab in Beaufort; learned to swim in Salter Path; was fired from her first job in Washington; was educated in Greenville and Durham; realized she wasn't a surfer or vegetarian in Corolla; and was a banker in Whiteville. Although she's lived the past 20 years in her beloved Lake Waccamaw, she calls New Bern home because that's where her mother and sister live.

Her new goal in life is one day to become one of those old women about whom the neighborhood children make up stories. "So far, so good!" she says. Lisa lives with her wonderdog, Aslan.

Printed in the United States
200267BV00001BB/160-438/A